How To Relieve Back Pain And Avoid Back Surgery

A Step-By-Step Guide Put Together by the Clinic Director of the Back Pain And Sciatica Clinic in Soquel, CA

DR. JOHN FALKENROTH, D.C.

DEDICATION

This is dedicated to the countless number of people in this world who suffer from back pain. I hope that this material that I put together will help back pain sufferers get back pain relief.

CONTENTS

ACKNOWLEDGMENTS

Thank you to all of my patients who have given me the privilege of trusting me with their health.

Thank you also to the thousands of patients who listened to my guidance. They have helped me gain the knowledge and the experience to further help others who suffer from back pain, neck pain and sciatica.

Thank you to all of the wonderful teachers throughout my life who gave me a solid educational foundation and instilled in me the love of learning.

Finally, I'd like to thank my family – my wife Estrella and my children James, Kevin and Starlyn – for their love and support.

SPECIAL NOTE

The information contained in this guide is solely advisory, and should not be substituted for medical advice. Any and all health care concerns, decisions, and actions must be done through the advice and counsel of a healthcare professional who is familiar with your updated medical history. We cannot be held responsible for actions you may take without a thorough exam or appropriate referral. If your condition is so severe that you have symptoms that prompt immediate surgical consideration such as loss of bladder and/or bowel control, etc., please get immediate medical care for your condition. Also understand that your results will vary. By following the information contained in this guide, you realize that you are doing so at your own risk and knowingly waive all rights to make any legal claims against Dr. John Falkenroth, D.C. or Back Pain & Sciatica Clinic or any site and/or site affiliates that this information may appear on.

1 WHAT CAUSES BACK PAIN

Back pain can be very debilitating. You must arm yourself with important information that you need to know to help make sure your condition does not become permanent and irreversible. Let's first go over what may be causing your back pain.

There are 3 main causes of back pain:
1. Mechanical
2. Nerve root pain
3. "Red Flags" or serious conditions.

Most low back conditions belong to the first group. Below is a partial list of conditions that belong to each of the three categories above.

Mechanical low back pain: causes of mechanical low back pain include lumbar and sacroiliac (SI) sprains, lumbar muscle strains, facet syndrome, degenerative disc disease and/or injury to the disc without nerve pinch, osteoarthritis (this can affect different parts of the spine), spinal instability, spondylolysis and/or spondylolisthesis, and more.

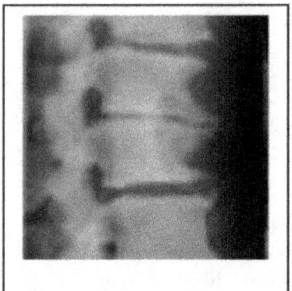

Here's an x-ray of a spine with a lot of problems... osteoarthritis, degenerative disc disease, etc. This person is probably having back pain now... or will have back pain in the future. Don't let your condition get this bad.

For mechanical low back pain, the pain pattern is usually localized to the low back and may spread into the buttocks, hips and thighs…but rarely extends past the knee. Usually, there is NO numbness or weakness in the leg or foot because that symptom suggests a spinal nerve pinch.

Nerve root pain: can result from a herniated disc, central or lateral spinal stenosis (usually caused by a combination of things including Degenerative Disc Disease) , arthritis, and/or calcification of ligaments near the nerve. These can be managed very successfully without surgery but the careful monitoring of numbness, muscle weakness, and treatment satisfaction is important.

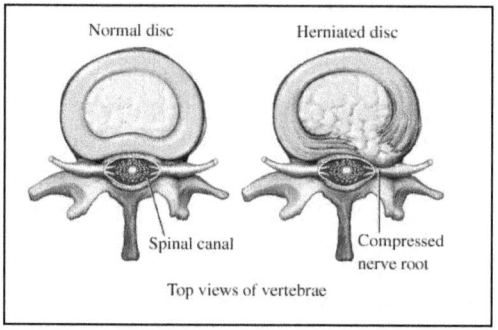

The above picture shows how a herniated disc can pinch a nerve.

Red Flags: These are the potentially dangerous conditions such as cancer, fracture, infections, and Cauda Equina Syndrome (spinal cord pinch creating bowel and/or bladder weakness). Referred pain from organs may be included here as well. As you can see, these carry potentially deadly consequences and require immediate referral and specialty management.

The majority of patients suffering from low back pain fall into the first two categories, and the HISTORY can tell us a lot.

If your low back pain stays mostly in your low back but sometimes spreads into your buttocks or thigh without numbness or weakness in your leg… and feels better with leaning forward or curling up in a ball, your back pain is most likely from a mechanical cause.

If there is numbness, tingling, and/or weakness in your leg to the foot and bending over hurts, your back pain is most likely from a disc problem… like a bulged disc or a herniated disc… with a nerve pinch. In

2

addition to back pain, you may also develop a condition known as sciatica.

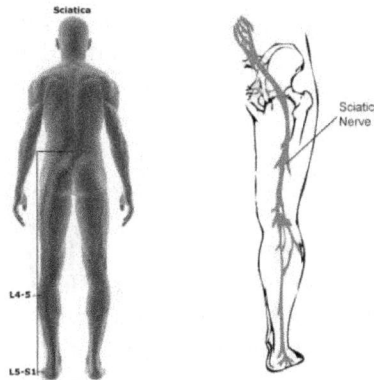

The figure above shows the pain/numbness/tingling pattern that people with sciatica commonly feel.

If there is unexplained weight loss, a past history of cancer, non-responding low back pain to treatment, sleep interruptions, and age >50 years old, your back pain may be caused by a more serious condition and further tests are needed.

Besides injuries to your back… and diseases that affect your spine, here are other common causes of back pain:

1. **MATTRESS:** Which type of mattress is best? The "short answer": there is no single mattress (style or type) for all people, primarily due to body type, size, gender, and what "feels good." TRY laying on a variety of mattresses (for several minutes on your back and sides) and check out the difference between coiled, inner springs, foam (of different densities), air, waterbeds, etc. The thickness of a mattress can vary from 7 to 18 inches (~17-45 cm) deep. Avoid mattresses that feel like you're sleeping in a hammock! A "good" mattress should maintain your natural spinal curves when lying on your sides or back (avoid sleeping on your stomach). Try placing a pillow between your knees and "hug" a pillow when side sleeping, as it can act like a "kick stand" and prevent you from rolling onto your stomach. If your budget is tight, you can "cheat" by placing a piece of plywood between the mattress and box spring as a short-term fix.

2. **SHOES:** Look at the bottom of the shoes that you normally wear and check out the "wear pattern." If you have worn out soles or heels, you

are way overdue for a new pair or a "re-sole" by your local shoe cobbler. If you have uneven wear and tear pattern between your right and left shoes, you may have a muscle imbalance... or a functional short leg, and/or collapsed arches in your feet. My patients that have these respond well when I fit them for their very own custom orthotics.

If you work on your feet, then it's very important that your feet get proper support for both managing and preventing low back pain.

3. **DIET:** A poor diet leads to obesity, which is a MAJOR cause of low back pain. Consider the Paleo or Mediterranean Diet and STAY AWAY from fast food! Identify the two or three "food abuses" you have embraced and eliminate them – things with empty calories like soda, ice cream, chips... you get the picture! Keeping your BMI (Body Mass Index) between 20 and 25 is the goal. Positive "side-effects" include increased longevity, better overall health, and an improved quality of life.

4. **EXERCISE:** The most effective self-help approach to low back pain management is exercise. Studies show that those who exercise regularly hurt less, see doctors less, have a higher quality of life, and just feel better. Plus, exercise helps keep your weight in check. Later in this book, we'll cover specific exercises for your back.

5. **POSTURE:** Another important "self-help" trick of the trade is to avoid sitting slumped over with an extreme forward head carriage position. Remember that every inch your head pokes forward places an additional ten pounds of load on your upper back muscles to keep your head upright... and sitting slumped increases the load on your entire back!

6. **OFFICE CHAIR:** Because of vast differences between people's height, weight, body type, and preference, it's difficult — if not impossible — to find a one-size-fits-all solution when it comes to office chairs! In the ideal world, the option to sit, stand, walk, and stretch as needed would be perfect but this simply is not reality. Low back pain from sitting is common due to the excess pressure it places on the joints and discs (the "shock-absorbers" of the spine). Here are some remedies: 1) Find a chair that FITS YOU. 2) Get up and move around at least once every hour (set a timer as a reminder). 3) Place your computer monitor directly in front of you and put your keyboard and mouse in a position so that your elbows bend only 90°. 4) Keep your feet on the floor at your desk (use an upside down box if your legs

don't touch the floor). 5) Perform "in the chair" stretches when your timer goes off and get up, take a break and move around.

7. **BODY TYPE:** We've discussed obesity as an obvious cause of back pain, but other factors are important as well. A very common cause of back pain for women is breast size. Big breasts add additional stress on the back and shoulders… wear a supportive bra if you have this issue.

8. **SHOULDER BAGS:** Back pain can be caused and/or made worse by a heavy purse, bag, briefcase, and even a thick wallet in the back pocket. To keep your eyes level, your body has to compensate and assume a less-than-ideal posture that may place unnecessary stress on your back. So before leaving the house today, CLEAN OUT your bag and put your wallet in a front pocket and lessen the load on your spine.

9. **SMOKING:** Smoking can reduce the amount of oxygen that reaches your cells, which can cause them to function at a less than optimal state. Maybe you've heard that a conscientious back surgeon will NEVER operate on a smoker's back due to both the prolonged healing time and the subsequent bad outcomes. So in addition to giving your heart, lungs, and those around you a break, if you want your lower back to heal, STOP SMOKING. Studies also show that smokers are TWICE as likely to develop low back pain compared to non-smokers… so quit. Better yet, DON'T START in the first place.

10. **STRESS AND DEPRESSION:** Remember, "health" is a balance between structure, chemistry, and mental factors. Stress increases muscle tightness and alters posture in a way that can lead to or worsen existing low back pain. Exercise, meditate, eat smart, and resolve your differences with family members and friends to minimize this problem… and get help when you need it.

11. **ERGONOMICS:** How we "fit" into our job, lifting properly, workstation set up, work pace, and work stressors ALL play into low back pain management. Have an assessment to see if you have proper ergonomics at your job. If you notice that your back hurts at work, you may not have proper ergonomics… or you're not taking enough breaks to relax your back… or you have a job that's not back-friendly. One common mistake young people make is doing manual jobs that are hard on the back. When you're young, you feel strong and flexible, but certain jobs make you prone to back injuries… and you'll usually feel the damage you've done to your back as you get older.

2 HOW BACK PAIN USUALLY STARTS AND HOW IT GETS WORSE

If we take things back one step further in figuring out the cause of your back pain... you may be surprised to know that your back pain may have started as abnormal movement or abnormal alignment of the bones in your spine... specifically in your low back.

This abnormal alignment and movement created uneven wear and tear on your spine... like the uneven wear and tear on your car tires when they're misaligned.

In the beginning, you may have noticed a clicking or a cracking sound when you moved your back... especially in a certain direction. This is because the misaligned part of your spine was probably rubbing abnormally against other parts.

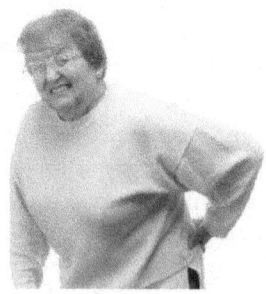

You may have also noticed your low back muscles feeling STIFF... especially in the morning.

You may have found yourself massaging your back or trying to stretch your low back throughout the day.

**Studies suggest that the longer
your spinal misalignments go uncorrected,
the GREATER your risk.**

If your back didn't get treated properly, it would have gotten worse.

Unfortunately, uncorrected spinal misalignments will usually advance to abnormal spinal conditions such as Spinal Arthritis, Bulged Discs or Herniated Discs, Degenerative Joint Disease or Spinal Stenosis. Any of these conditions can lead to back pain... and/or sciatica.

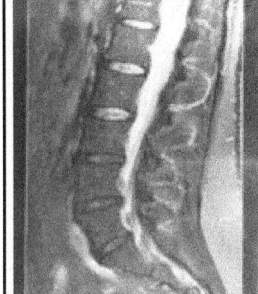

Notice the herniated discs in this lumbar spinal MRI. Bulged Discs and Herniated Discs like these can cause severe pinching of the delicate nerve roots that make up your sciatic nerve causing Sciatica.

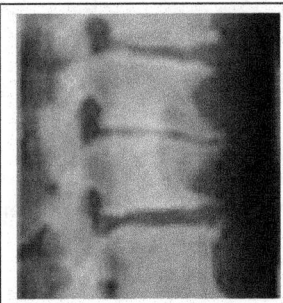

If you develop Spinal Arthritis or Degenerative Joint Disease in your low back, the bone spurs that you'll get from this condition may also pinch your sciatic nerve roots causing Sciatica.

Before developing severe back pain or sciatica, you may have felt a sharp pain, a dull ache or stiffness in your low back... for days, months or even years.

If your low back condition didn't get treated properly, your minor low back pain may have progressed to a sharp shooting pain, burning pain or numbness down your butt, back of your thigh, or back of your leg or foot... a condition known as sciatica.

Usually, sciatica symptoms are only on one leg or one thigh or one foot. But it's possible to have sciatica on both legs, thighs or feet.

For some people, their back pain and/or sciatica comes and goes.

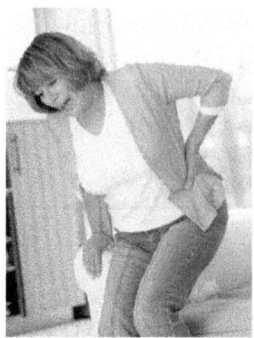

If you pay close attention, you'll notice that your pain, numbness or tingling is worse than the last episode.

In the beginning, your back pain may have been more of an annoyance versus being debilitating. But your nerve pain and numbness can quickly become serious and debilitating after doing a MINOR activity such as sleeping the wrong way, sitting the wrong way, picking up an object from the ground... or lifting an object.

As your condition gets worse, your pinched nerve will slowly die.

Because of this, you'll lose function. Without proper nerve input, your back, butt, thigh, leg and/or foot muscles on the side of your symptoms will get smaller and weaker.

Your affected muscles may also develop scar tissues... similar to the gristle that you see in a cheap cut of meat.

Your lost muscle mass and lost muscle strength will make it more difficult for you to climb stairs or walk up hills.

In the beginning, it's harder to notice the muscle loss in your back, butt, thigh, leg or foot. Have someone look at these areas and see if they notice muscle loss or a difference in muscle mass between the two sides.

If you lose muscle mass in your foot, you may notice that your shoe on the side of your symptom will be looser than the other side.

Because of your muscle imbalance, you may also notice that one of your hips is higher than the other hip… or that one of your legs is shorter than the other… a functional short leg.

This can cause uneven wear patterns on your shoes.

Look at the bottom of the shoes that you normally wear. Do you see uneven wear and tear patterns between your right shoe and your left shoe?

You may also notice being more clumsy… for example, tripping more often. Besides losing muscle mass and strength, you'll also most likely LOSE normal range of motion and flexibility in your low back spine… and maybe in your leg and foot.

A lot of people can deal with the nagging nerve pain or numbness… especially when it comes and goes. But it's a lot harder for people to deal with the loss of function that comes later when their back pain or Nerve Impingement Syndrome doesn't get fixed.

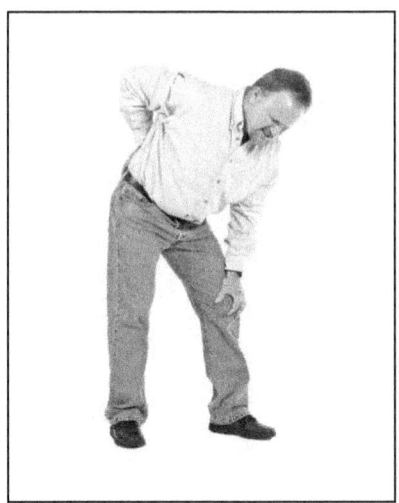

If caught and treated early, most back pain can be fixed without much loss of function.

However, untreated back pain that progresses to the advanced degenerative stages almost always results in PERMANENT loss of function that will affect your activities of daily living… including your job and your hobbies.

For example, most of us take for granted being able to sit in the car and drive. But, if your back pain gets worse, just the act of sitting in the car can be excruciatingly painful… making driving dangerous for you and for those around you.

The sooner you receive proper treatment for your back pain, the better your chances of a FULL AND COMPLETE RECOVERY.

Of course it's best if you consult a back pain expert who can find the cause of your problem and help you get relief.

3 THE ROAD TO RECOVERY... THINGS YOU SHOULD AVOID DOING

What exactly can you do to get back pain relief?

You can get back surgery... or you can try the following 7 non-surgical ways to help you get back pain relief... and hopefully help you avoid surgery.

I have a chiropractic clinic in Soquel, CA. After 16 years in practice, I've helped over 3,500 patients and many of them suffered from back pain.

The advice that you're about to get are the same advice that I give to my patients who have back pain.

Before you follow my suggestions in this book, be sure to consult with your doctor who is familiar with your medical history and current condition and get their okay. After you get their okay, here's what I advise you do...

If you have back pain, one thing you should AVOID is carrying your wallet or cell phone in the back pocket of your pants.

STOP doing this...

It may be causing your back pain and/or sciatica... especially if your problem is on the same side where you carry your wallet or cell phone. Carrying your cell phone or wallet in the back pocket of your pants can irritate your Piriformis… which can irritate your sciatic nerve under your piriformis. It can also create an abnormal alignment in your back and create postural imbalance.

Another thing to AVOID is assuming the worst position for your back.

Here's the #1 back position to avoid: BENDING over… while TWISTING your back… while REACHING for an object… while LIFTING or PULLING that object.

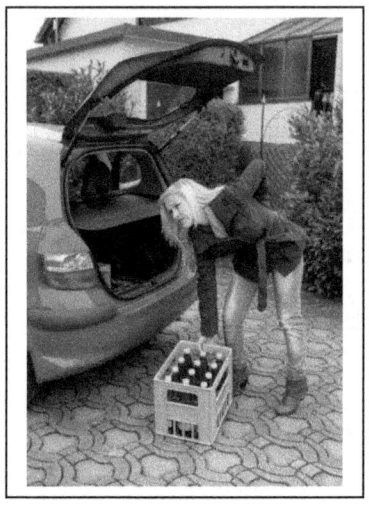

This combo move is a KILLER to your low back joints, muscles, ligaments and discs.

Many kids and adults do this without knowing how bad this position is for your back. When you're young and limber, you may be able to assume this back position without much pain afterward.

As you get older, you'll notice stiffness or pain in your low back while assuming the above position… or soon after.

If the object that you're reaching for and lifting or pulling is heavy… your back is in BIG TROUBLE. You may even hear a "pop" in your back when you injure your discs. This popping sound is BAD NEWS.

Besides avoiding the worst position for your back... you should also avoid the back positions that make your back pain worse.

When it comes to back pain... NO pain, NO gain is NOT a good rule. Some people feel like the pain is creating a good stretch in their low back.

Not so... if you're putting your back in a position that makes your back pain worse, you're probably doing more HARM than GOOD.

Avoiding positions that make your back pain worse is a simple RULE OF THUMB that you should follow. Following this rule of thumb will help relieve your back pain and speed up your recovery.

Ignoring this rule of thumb, will make your back pain worse and will make your back pain treatment NOT as effective.

The painful back positions to AVOID are different for different people.

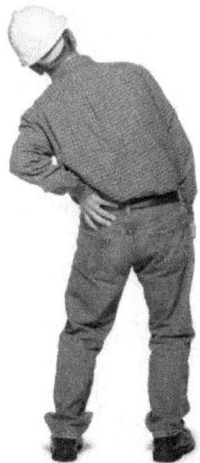

**Depending on what the painful back positions
are for you... tells a back pain expert A LOT
about what may be wrong with your back.**

What about moving your back in different positions to loosen up your back? If done correctly, it's good to stretch and loosen up your back. But, don't move your back in the directions that cause pain... SHARP PAIN.

Knowing this information and following this advice can mean the difference between getting better and becoming a candidate for back surgery.

Avoiding painful back positions is a "no brainer" for some people. But for others, it's very helpful in stopping their spinal damage... and preventing further injury to their spine. With this foundation, you're on your way to getting better.

Remember, avoid bending over... while TWISTING your back... while REACHING for an object... while LIFTING or PULLING that object.

Also, take note of the activities that you do that require you to do this BAD combo move... and either avoid these activities or change them.

Another thing to avoid is sitting too long.

The chronic habit of sitting too long puts a lot of pressure on your low back discs... dehydrating them... causing degenerative disc disease... which can lead to bulging discs and/or herniated discs.

Also, sitting too long can irritate your Piriformis. An irritated Piriformis muscle can lead to an irritated sciatic nerve... which can lead to sciatica.

As much as possible, minimize your sitting time. But, this might be easier said than done. Maybe your job or daily life requires you to SIT for long periods of time.

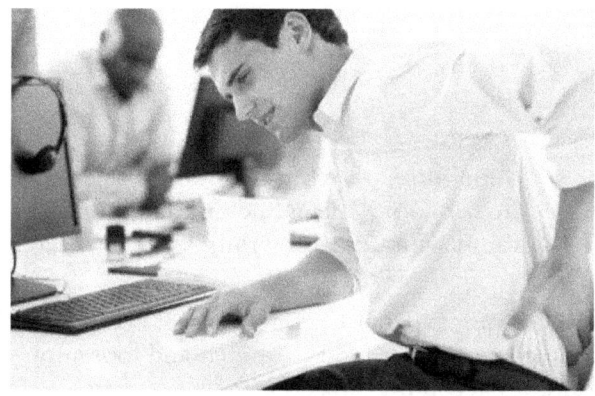

**Prolonged sitting is BRUTAL to your spinal discs...
especially to your low back or lumbar discs.**

If you absolutely have to sit for long periods during your waking hours, there is one simple gadget that you can buy to take some LOAD OFF your low back discs while you sit. This gadget will also help you maintain a proper posture while you sit.

What is this gadget?

It's a back rest. Not just any back rest... a good back rest. There are many back rests being sold today. Find the one that works best for you... the one that helps you keep proper posture while sitting down. If you need our help finding a good back rest for you, just ask us. We've tried many back rests, and we have a couple that we recommend to our patients.

Sit with this back rest on your chair and see how much easier it is to keep proper posture while you sit. Your low back discs will thank you.

4 THE PROPER STANDING AND SITTING POSTURE FOR BACK PAIN RELIEF

Now that we've told you what back positions to avoid... you should be wondering what the best back position is. Let's now discuss proper back posture.

According to Nobel Prize winner Dr. Hans Selye, M.D., *"The beginning of the disease process starts with postural distortions."*☐

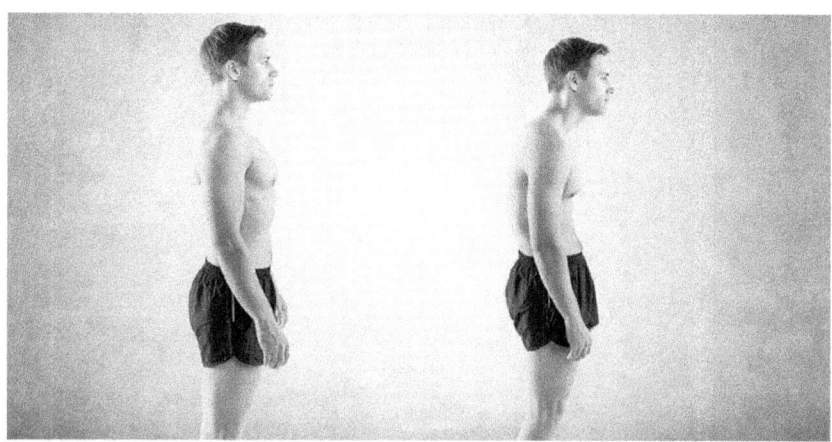

The picture on the left shows proper standing posture.
The picture on the right shows improper standing posture.

Find a mirror right now. Look at your posture in the mirror. Are your shoulders even? Are your hips even? How can you tell if your hips are even?

Use your hands to feel your lowest ribs on each side of your body. Move your hands down until you feel the top of your pelvic bone. Look at where your hands are in the mirror. Are they even... or is one hand higher than the other hand?

Now have someone look at you from the side. Is your head sitting straight above your neck and in line with your shoulders?

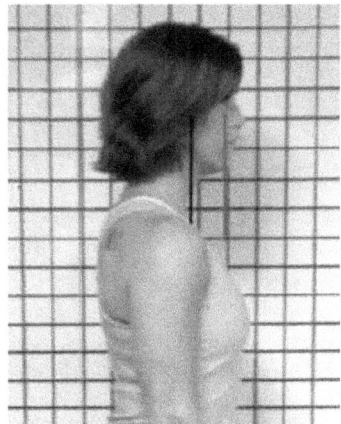

Or do you hold your head forward in front of your shoulders like in the picture above of bad forward head posture? With proper posture, your ear opening should be in line with your shoulder.

Poor posture is associated with asymmetries in motion, leading to accelerated degenerative spinal joint pathology that will, in time, adversely affect the nervous system. (Koch et al, 2002)

Since we spend a lot of time sitting, what's the best sitting posture?

Put your head in neutral position... looking straight ahead... not looking up and not looking down. Make sure your head is in line with your neck, shoulders and low back. This is the best sitting posture.

Can you COMFORTABLY keep this position for 30 MINUTES?

If not, you may have a problem in your neck or back that's preventing you from having good posture. Problems like spinal misalignments, spinal arthritis, muscle weakness, muscle spasms, etc. All of these problems SHOULD be corrected right away.

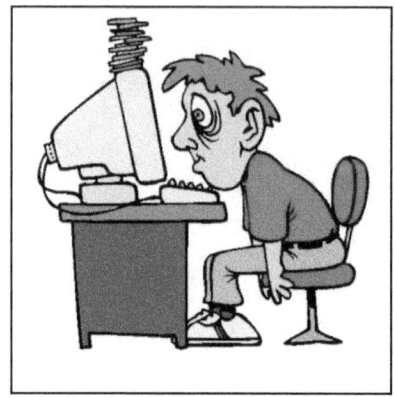

Bad sitting posture...

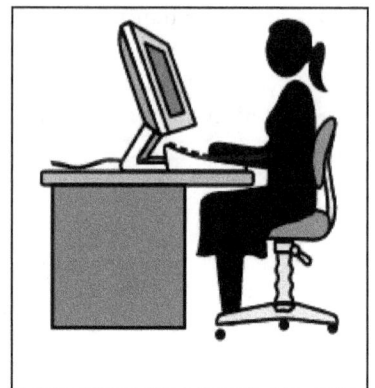

Good sitting posture...

Good posture is not just good for your back... it's also good for the rest of your body... and for your overall health and well-being.

Let me show you just how important good posture is to your health. Let's test how posture affects your lung capacity and LUNG HEALTH.

1. Sit on a chair.
2. Take a deep breath.
3. Assume the best posture position for your neck and back.
4. Take a deep breath.
5. Now slouch as much as you can or assume a bad posture.
6. Take a deep breath.

Could you tell the difference between your lung's ability to get enough oxygen when you sit with a GOOD posture versus when you sit with a BAD posture?

Every part of your body relies on getting enough oxygen to stay healthy.. function well... and to NOT get DISEASE.

If you continue to sit or stand with a bad posture that minimizes the flow of oxygen to the rest of your body parts that need oxygen... it's just a

18

matter of time before your oxygen-deprived body parts will break down... and disease will set in.

Here again is Dr. Selye's quote:

"The beginning of the disease process starts with postural distortions." This statement seems far-fetched at first. BUT... I hope you realize now that it makes sense. After all, Dr. Hans Selye, M.D. is a Nobel Prize winner. He MUST know what he's talking about.

5 DO THIS SIMPLE ACTIVITY TO RELIEVE BACK PAIN

Walking is one often overlooked activity that can relieve back pain. Walking is ESSENTIAL to your healing and recovery... a simple yet powerful activity. Walking is a fantastic way to exercise your back and make it strong and flexible.

Walk a few steps right now with your arms lightly swinging by your side. Did you feel your spinal muscles, ligaments and joints moving? You may not have felt your joints and ligaments moving, but you should have felt the muscles along your spine moving.

Try it again... and don't forget the gentle arm swing.

Walking creates a POWERFUL PUMP in your spine that helps pump fluids and nutrients in and out of your spinal joints... including your spinal discs.

Walking is a good way to maintain circulation in your spine. Walking will also help prevent stiffness of your muscles and keep them from getting too spastic.

Also, if you pay close attention while you walk, you'll notice that your spinal muscles move in a synchronized way... where they alternate between stretching and contracting... a very elegant movement that's an absolute MUST for keeping your spinal muscles relaxed, flexible, strong and healthy.

Walk again... with a gentle arm swing... and see if you can feel this synchronized movement of your back muscles.

So, whenever you're able... WALK. But, don't overdo it. Too much of anything... including something that's good for you... is NOT good.

If you're like most people with back pain, you're probably NOT walking too much. Squeeze in more walking time during your daily life to help relieve your back pain.

If you're not used to walking... or if your back pain is severe... you may have to start walking on FLAT, SOFT surfaces such as grass or trails first before you tackle walking on hills... or on a harder surface like pavement.

Also, if you're like most people with back pain, you may be out of shape. You can even START walking inside your house. If you feel the need to rest or to sit down after walking some distance... sit down and rest.

If you have someone you can walk with, walk with them. Walking with a partner is not only good for your back, but it will also be good for your emotional health.

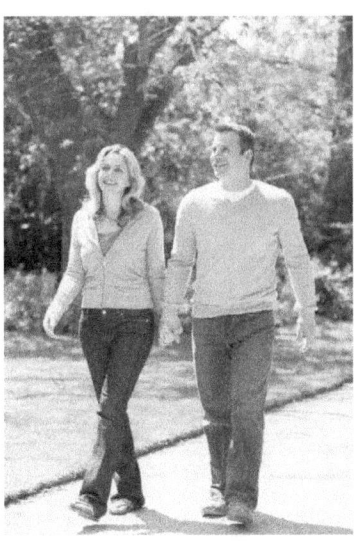

Take a healthy friend with you who can help you in case you need extra assistance.

21

If you're able, walk outside so that you can get the benefit of getting extra oxygen in your system. Oxygen is also VITAL to your healing and recovery.

Make sure there are rest stops along the way for you to sit on in case you need to rest. If you sit on the ground, it may be very difficult and very painful for you to get back up.

If walking makes your back pain unbearable, you should talk to your doctor for other things you can do to keep your lower back and legs moving.

If your doctor says that it's okay for you to do some walking, don't overdo it. Do not go beyond your pain tolerance. Do not go beyond your fitness tolerance.

6 HOW MUCH WATER YOU SHOULD DRINK FOR YOUR CONDITION

How much water is adequate? Do you need 8 glasses of water a day... no matter how tall you are or how much you weigh?

Here's a different suggestion as far as proper fluid intake that takes your body size and activity level into account.

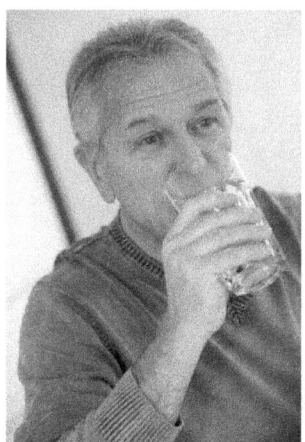

Divide your weight in half and the number you get is the amount of fluids in ounces (ozs.) that you should be drinking throughout the day.

For example, if you weigh 160 lbs... dividing 160 by 2 gives you 80... so you should drink about 80 ounces of water a day.

If you're more active during the day, you may need more water that day. Also, if the weather is hot, you may need more water.

Making sure you get enough fluids will help you recover from back pain. This is especially important for people with dehydrated spinal discs... which is often the case in people who suffer from back pain.

Water also helps flush inflammatory byproducts out of your system.

Just make sure you're drinking good quality fluids and not the kind that dehydrate you such as coffee, alcohol or sodas.

Also, you might notice that when you drink more water, you tend to use the bathroom more. This is usual for most people in the beginning when they increase their water intake. Soon, your body should adjust to your new hydration level.

You may also need less water... especially if you don't have an active lifestyle. Too much of anything including something that's good for you such as water, is NOT good.

Get enough water, but not too much.

7 SHOULD YOU USE ICE OR HEAT FOR YOUR BACK PAIN?

Ice your low back to help relieve your back pain. Ice is an anti-inflammatory agent... meaning it reduces inflammation or swelling.

Ice reduces congestion or PUSHES out of the injured area painful chemicals and fluids that build up when there's inflammation. Ice usually feels good... once the part that you're icing is numb... but because ice is cold, it may not feel good in the beginning.

Heat does the opposite of ice.

Heat PULLS fluids INTO an area. Unlike ice, heat feels good initially. But often, people who use heat on their low back say that it later made their back problem WORSE.

This is because the additional fluid build-up in an already inflamed or injured area is kind of like throwing gasoline on a fire.

Where *exactly* should you put the ice? Put the ice over the area of your low back that hurts.

If your low back pain is caused by a spastic, tight or irritated Piriformis muscle, ice the affected Piriformis.

If you have both low back problem and Piriformis muscle problem, ice BOTH your low back and your Piriformis.

25

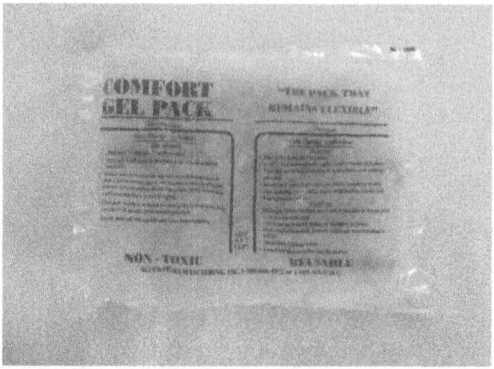

When using ice therapy... instead of using ice cubes, it's better to use the moldable ice packs like the one above with the gel-like material inside.

These moldable ice packs come in different sizes and quality. Part of your at-home first aid supply should be a good ice pack.

DON'T PUT THE ICE PACK DIRECTLY ON YOUR SKIN.

Instead, put a thin piece of clothing... like your t-shirt... or a thin towel between your skin and the ice pack. You can have a thicker barrier if you're too chilled when using just a t-shirt or a thin towel.

Also, DO NOT lie face down. Instead, ice your low back while you're lying face up or while you're sitting.

And how long exactly should you keep the ice on?

This really depends on your current condition and diagnosis. If you have a condition that is "uncomplicated," use the ice pack for 15-20 minutes every 3-4 hours.

WARNING: Before you use ice, make sure you don't have a vascular or a neurologic condition that makes it unsafe for you to use ice.

8 THE BACK PAIN EXERCISES THAT YOU SHOULD CONSIDER DOING

Stretching exercises work best when the cause of your back pain is from a tight or spastic muscle.

PROCEED WITH CAUTION WITH THESE EXERCISES.

If you don't know exactly which low back stretches and exercises to do, DON'T do any. Ignorance in this area can hurt you and can make your back pain worse

But... there are easy exercises that most people with back pain can safely do. If you feel SHARP PAIN in your low back... or anywhere... while doing any of these exercises, STOP immediately.

Many back problems can be relieved by back exercises. But if you're getting SHARP PAIN with any of the exercises that I'm about to cover, your back pain may be beyond this point.

You may have a serious condition that needs expert help.

WARNING: As a general rule, if your back pain is caused by a herniated disc or a bulged disc, DON'T do the exercises that require you to bend your torso forward. Also, DON'T do the exercises that require you to bend your leg(s) up.

If your back pain is caused by referred pain from an irritated low back spinal facet joint, DON'T do the exercises that require you to bend your torso backward.

Some of the exercises that I'll show you are advanced… so depending on how severe your back pain is… you may not be able to do all of these exercises.

Typically, when you do the exercises that are "BAD" for your specific condition, you'll notice that your back pain, and/or leg numbness and/or tingling will feel WORSE.

It's best to consult a back pain expert who can help you determine the cause of your back problem before you do any of these exercises.

Back Range of Motion Exercises:

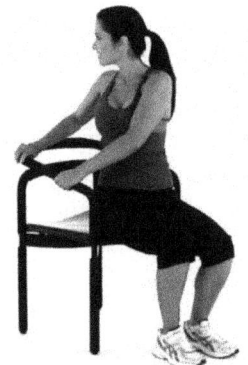 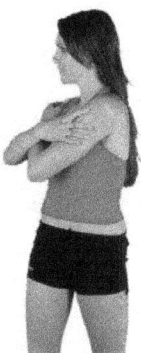

Do these stretches CAREFULLY. Don't move your back quickly… move it nice and slow. You can stretch your back while sitting or while standing.

While keeping your back straight, move your back forward. Then backward. Then left. Then right. Then move your upper body to look over your RIGHT shoulder. Then move your upper body to look over your LEFT shoulder.

If your back pain is caused by a herniated or bulged low back disc, you may find bending forward very painful… so DON'T bend forward.

You may also find bending to one side very painful… so DON'T bend to the side that's painful.

If you have an MRI, you can ask your doctor to show you the exact direction that your disc has herniated. Based on the location of your herniated disc, your doctor should be able to tell you which position(s) might make your back pain worse… and which position(s) might relieve your back pain.

If your herniated disc or bulged disc is severe, you may not find a comfortable position…all positions may hurt.

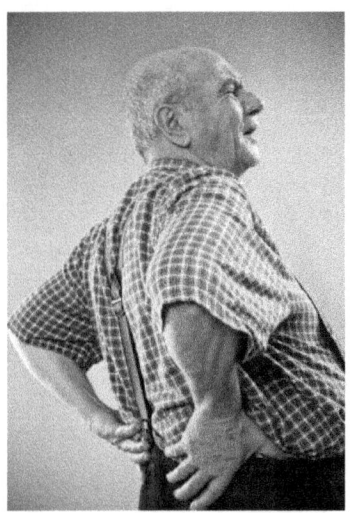

If your back pain is caused by a referred pain from an inflamed facet joint in your low back, you may find bending backward very painful… so DON'T bend backward.

Again, if you feel SHARP PAIN in your low back or anywhere while doing any of the above exercises, STOP immediately.

Other Back Exercises And Stretches:

Some of these will stretch your back and spine… some will help you keep proper posture… some will strengthen your core muscles.

We'll start with seated exercises, then standing, then lying down. If you have severe back pain, you may not be able to assume some of these positions… let alone do the exercises… so again, proceed carefully. Only do the exercises that you can comfortably do without getting sharp pain or without getting stuck in a painful position.

Seated Flexion

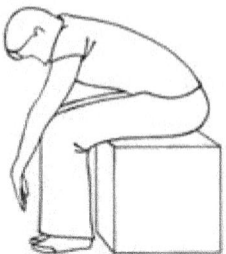

While sitting at the edge of a chair... suck your stomach in... slowly bend your upper body forward... bending vertebra by vertebra from the head down. Bend forward at the waist (not at the hips) to feel a stretch in your low back. Repeat.

Chin Protraction And Retraction:

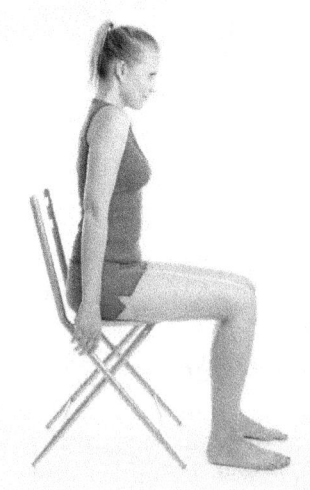

Sit with your head in neutral position – looking straight ahead. While keeping this neutral position, jut your chin forward... then retract your chin back. Repeat.

Pectoral Release:

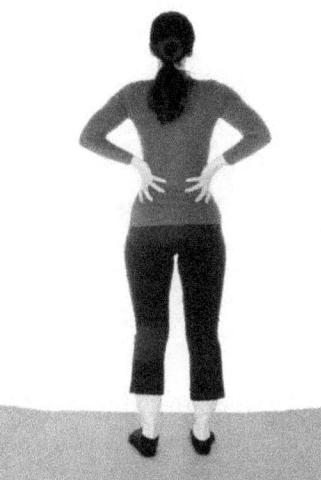

Stand up and put both your palms on your low back. Breathe in and raise your chest up while bringing your elbows toward each other behind your body. Hold... then exhale, feeling a release in the front of your chest and shoulders. Return to starting position. Repeat.

Forward Lunge:

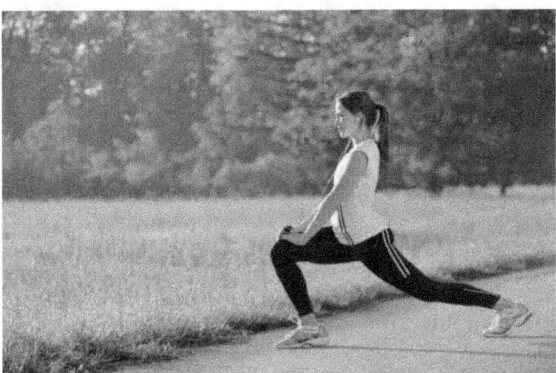

Stand with your feet shoulder width apart and toes pointing forward. Put one foot forward into a lunge position with your back foot staying up on your toes. While keeping your body upright and both hips in line, straighten out your back knee. You should feel a stretch in the front of your thigh and hip on the same side as your back foot. Repeat on the other side.

Prayer Stretch:

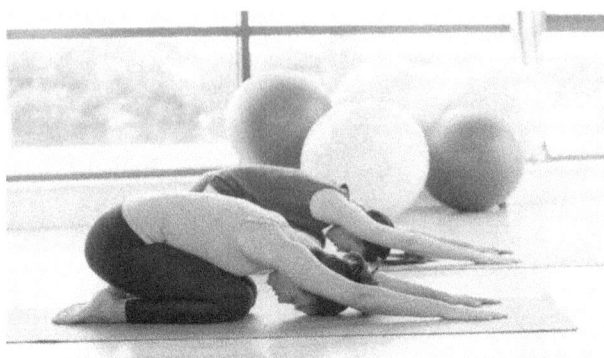

Kneel on the floor, reach both arms straight out in front along the floor. Move your upper body down so that your buttocks are resting on your heels. Go back to the starting position. Repeat.

Quadruped Arm Raises:

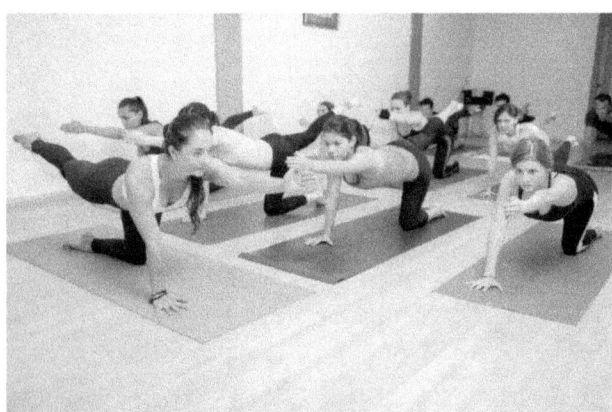

While on your hands and knees... and while maintaining abdominal hollow... and while keeping your back flat, slowly raise one of your arms out in front until it's parallel with the floor. Lower your raised arm to the floor. Repeat on the other side.

If you're able, you can also slowly lift up your leg opposite your raised arm until your leg is parallel to the floor. If you are going to also do this, lift up your leg the same time you lift up your arm.

Chest Raise/Airplane:

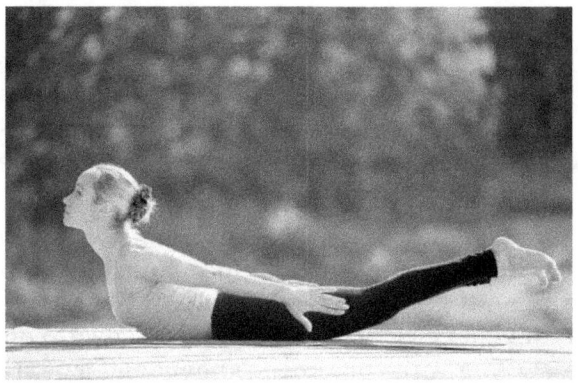

Lie on your stomach with your arms at your sides at 45° angle. Keep a slight chin tuck position... or don't look up. Squeeze your midback and raise your chest up off the floor. Hold. Go back to starting position. Repeat.

If you're able, turn your palm out so that your thumbs point to the ceiling. Also, if you're able, lift your feet off the ground when you lift your chest off the ground... you can also look up if you'd like.

Abdominal Hollow:

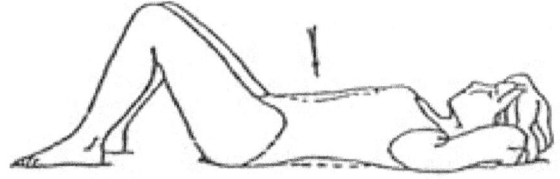

Tighten your abdomen by moving your belly button closer to your back. Repeat.

You can also tighten your abdomen while sitting or while standing. This means that you can do this exercise while you wait in line at stores or while you're waiting for someone.

Doing this simple exercise... often... can help strengthen your abdominal muscles... which can help relieve your back pain.

Knee To Chest:

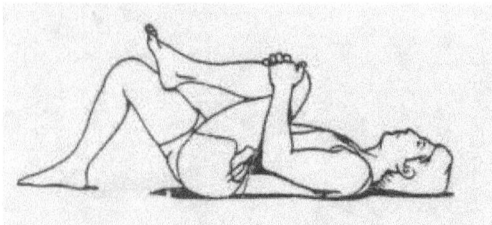 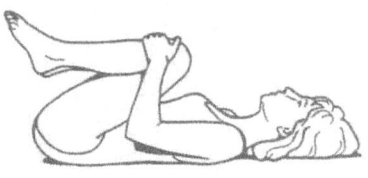

Lie down on your back with your legs bent. Bring one knee toward your chest... hold under the knee joint. Hold. Put your leg back to the starting position. Repeat on the other side. If you're able, bring both knees toward your chest at the same time. Repeat. You can also do this exercise starting with your knees unbent and legs straight.

You can use your hands to help keep your knees bent, but don't use your hands to help you stretch farther... you may "overstretch" and injure yourself.

Don't overdo this stretch... and don't hold your leg in the bent position too long.

With all of the back exercises and stretches that I discussed in this section, you're probably asking the following questions:

- How long should I hold each position?
- How many repetitions should I do?
- How many times a day should I do them?
- When should I do these exercises?

Let's start with how long you should hold each position. Start holding each position for 2-3 seconds. As you get stronger, you may be able to hold them longer... but don't overdo it.

How many repetitions should you do?

Do as many as you can comfortably handle... and again, don't overdo it! Start with 3-5 reps... less if you're not able to.

How many times a day should you do them?

Twice a day works well for most people. Also, it's best to do these exercises more often rather than do a lot of reps and/or long holds.

After you do the above exercises and stretches, you might feel sore in certain areas. Ice these areas... follow the icing instructions covered in the previous section.

When's the best time to do these exercises?

Do them at a time that works best for you. Also, they're so simple that if you feel your back starting to hurt or starting to tighten up... stop what you're doing and do these exercises.

DON'T do these exercises first thing in the morning. Your muscles and ligaments won't be warmed up... you'll be more prone to injury.

Also, don't do these exercises when you're EXHAUSTED... your muscles and ligaments won't have as much strength to protect your joints if you overstretch.

9 HOW TO KEEP YOUR SPINE ALIGNED AND MOVING PROPERLY

Since misaligned spinal joints and/or spinal joints that don't move properly can cause back pain… or make back pain worse… make sure to keep your proper spinal alignment and motion.

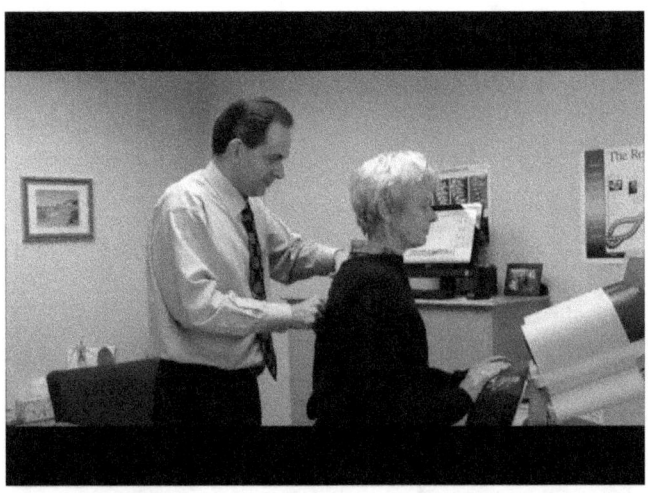

You should see a chiropractor who can check your spine for proper alignment and motion.

This will not only help relieve your back pain, but keeping your spinal bones and joints aligned and moving properly will help prevent future problems from showing up later.

How?

Each bone and joint in your spine is connected to each other... especially the ones directly above and directly below each spinal bone/joint.

When you have spinal misalignment or abnormal spinal motion, the joints above and below the problem joint will need to compensate to keep the alignment and motion of your spine as close to normal as possible.

These joints will start to have problems if they have to keep compensating... then the bones and joints around them will also need to compensate causing problems in these areas.

If not stopped, you'll have a vicious cycle of spinal joint degeneration happening up and down your spine. You may notice that over time, the joints above and below the initial problem area will also develop degenerative joint problems.

This is why people with low back problem often also end up experiencing neck problems.

Different chiropractors use different chiropractic treatment techniques and different approaches to keep your spinal bones aligned and your spinal joints moving properly.

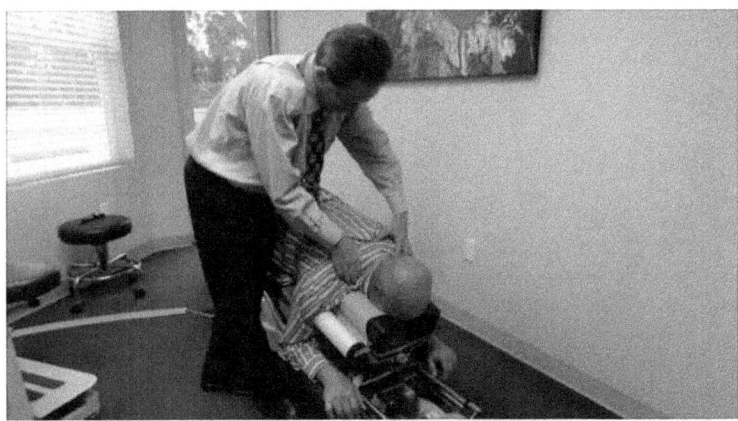

Some chiropractors use traditional hands-on treatments like this one above that I use at my clinic.

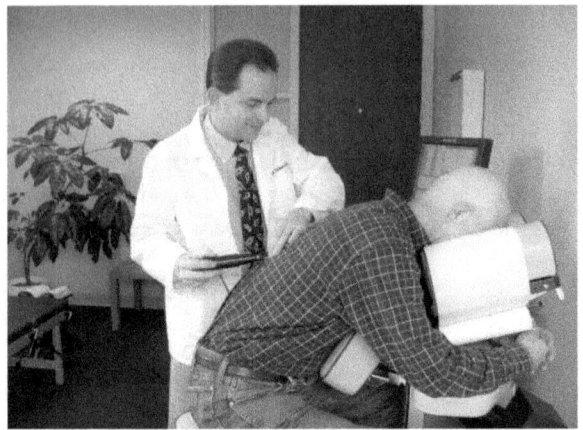

Some chiropractors use instrument-guided treatment like the one above. I use this on my patients who don't like their necks or backs cracked, popped or twisted.

Some chiropractors use BOTH the traditional hands-on treatments and also instrument-guided treatments.

Find a chiropractor who uses a treatment style that works best for you.

10 MODERN TREATMENTS THAT HELP RELIEVE BACK PAIN

If your back pain is from a bulged disc or a herniated disc, there are modern machines that can gently stretch your low back… and relieve your pinched nerves or nerve roots.

Below is an example of a modern back traction machine.

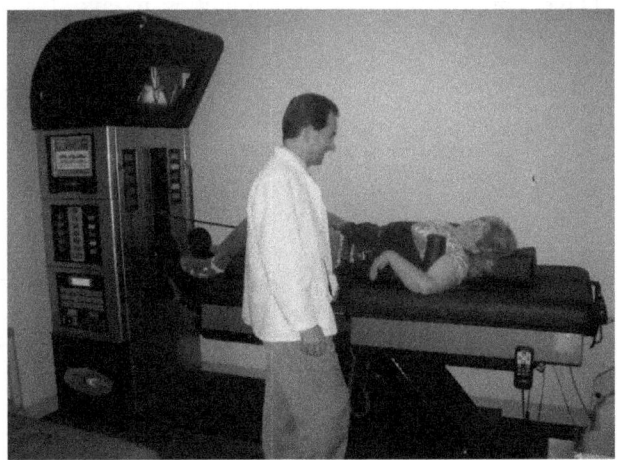

Being on this machine is so EASY and RELAXING that most of my patients that use this machine take a short nap during their session. Plus, a lot of them get excellent results.

Some of these stretching machines get impressive results. The one in the previous page was designed by doctors, scientists and engineers. The goal of these stretching machines is to gently stretch your low back and release any pinched nerve and/or nerve roots... and some can help rehydrate your dehydrated low back discs.

Be careful when choosing which stretching machines to try. Some may help you. Some may make your condition worse.

There are stretching devices that some people with back pain use that stretch their backs at home... unsupervised by a health care practitioner. Be very careful with these at-home back stretching devices.

You may do more harm than good. Consult your doctor before trying one of these at-home devices.

No matter what back pain treatment or device you try... don't lose hope. Many people with back pain have successfully overcome their condition... or at least made their back pain manageable without much loss of function... allowing them to continue to work and/or continue to enjoy their favorite activities and hobbies.

Aren't you tired of constantly trying to find a comfortable pain-free position? Have you LIMITED your activities to avoid getting seriously hurt?

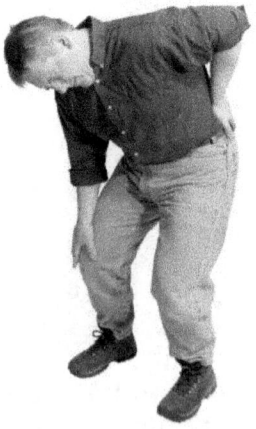

**Is it getting harder to stand or to sit for a long time?
Especially on a hard surface? You probably lost
so much function and flexibility already.**

How much more flexibility and function can you stand to lose?

You may have decided to live with your back pain or your leg/foot pain, tingling or numbness. After treating hundreds of patients with back pain, I know that back pain can progress from a manageable pain to a painfully debilitating pain… sometimes overnight.

After accidentally bending or twisting your back in the "wrong direction," you may feel that instant knife stabbing pain in your low back or leg… compounded by a severe low back muscle spasm… that feels like a giant wrench clamping your back… freezing you in your tracks… while your blood pressure and pulse rate skyrocket.

Get help now before this happens to you.

If after you follow my advice in this book, your back pain is not MUCH BETTER… you may have a condition that's beyond something that you can correct at home.

There are a lot of good doctors around that can help you with your back pain. If you live in Santa Cruz County, California… or if you find yourself in this area, come by my clinic… The Back Pain And Sciatica Clinic… to see if I can help you with your back pain. Below is my contact information:

Back Pain And Sciatica Clinic
Dr. John Falkenroth, D.C.
2959 Park Ave., Suite F
Soquel, CA 95073
(831) 475-8600
www.BackPainAndSciaticaClinic.com

I hope that the information that I shared with you will help relieve your back pain. I wish you the best of luck in finding the back pain relief that you're looking for.

Thank you for your time.

ABOUT THE AUTHOR

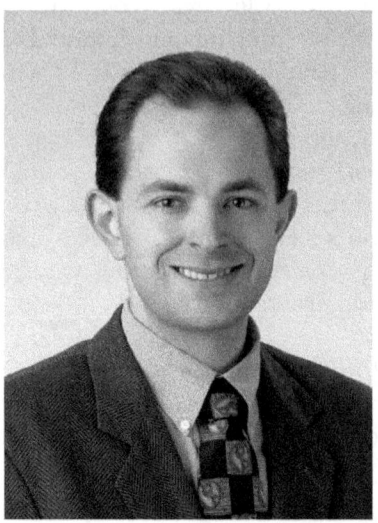

Dr. John Falkenroth, D.C. is the Clinic Director at the Back Pain And Sciatica Clinic in Soquel, California, USA. After over 16 years practicing chiropractic, Dr. Falkenroth has helped over 3,500 patients... many of them suffered from back pain, neck pain and sciatica.

Prior to attending chiropractic school, Dr. Falkenroth attended the University of California at Davis... where he earned a Bachelor of Science degree in Physiology in 1994.

While studying human physiology at the University of California at Davis, Dr. Falkenroth realized that pressure or impingement on the spinal nerve roots that exit the spine can negatively affect a person's health.

With this realization, Dr. Falkenroth decided to help others by becoming an expert in treating back pain, neck pain and sciatica.

To complement his excellent physiology background from UC Davis, Dr. Falkenroth decided to go to Davenport, Iowa, USA to attend the 100+ year old top-rated chiropractic college in the world – Palmer College – where he graduated *summa cum laude*.

Go to the website www.BackPainAndSciaticaClinic.com for more back pain relief tips. You can also call Dr. Falkenroth's office in Soquel at (831) 475-8600.

www.ingramcontent.com/pod-product-compliance
Lightning Source LLC
Chambersburg PA
CBHW071005180526
45168CB00003B/1289